T0332711

Skin Diseases of Cattle in the Tropics

Skin Diseases of Cattle in the Tropics

A Guide to Diagnosis and Treatment

Mohamed E. Hamid
Faculty of Veterinary Medicine, University of Khartoum,
Khartoum North, Sudan

AMSTERDAM • BOSTON • HEIDELBERG • LONDON
NEW YORK • OXFORD • PARIS • SAN DIEGO
SAN FRANCISCO • SINGAPORE • SYDNEY • TOKYO
Academic Press is an imprint of Elsevier

ELSEVIER

Academic Press is an imprint of Elsevier
125 London Wall, London EC2Y 5AS, UK
525 B Street, Suite 1800, San Diego, CA 92101-4495, USA
50 Hampshire Street, 5th Floor, Cambridge, MA 02139, USA
The Boulevard, Langford Lane, Kidlington, Oxford OX5 1GB, UK

British Library Cataloguing-in-Publication Data
A catalogue record for this book is available from the British Library

Library of Congress Cataloging-in-Publication Data
A catalog record for this book is available from the Library of Congress

ISBN: 978-0-12-811054-6

For Information on all Academic Press publications
visit our website at http://www.elsevier.com/

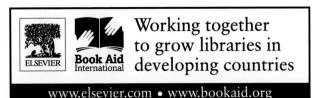

Working together
to grow libraries in
developing countries

www.elsevier.com • www.bookaid.org

Publisher: Sara Tenney
Acquisition Editor: Kristi Gomez
Editorial Project Manager: Pat Gonzalez
Production Project Manager: Kiruthika Govindaraju
Cover Designer: MPS

Typeset by MPS Limited, Chennai, India

CONTENTS

INTRODUCTION

Skin Diseases of Cattle in the Tropics: Guide to Diagnosis and Treatment is a clinical and practical guide to help field veterinarians, veterinary students, and technicians to make appropriate and differential diagnoses. It provides quizzes of clinical cases and demonstrates more than 100 images of characteristic lesions and laboratory findings of major skin diseases and diseases with skin manifestations prevalent in tropical areas notably the Sub-Saharan African countries. This self-learning and easy-to-use instructional guide, the only one of its kind in the field of veterinary medicine, provides, firstly, the condition (as a quiz); followed by its laboratory diagnosis; then answers to the quiz and a summary of the disease.

The book was proposed in order to make the subject accessible for practicing veterinarians and useful for those who have neither seen nor had the chance to see such diseases in the field or clinics. Such diseases are important not only in the tropics but can be encountered in many countries in subtropical and temperate zones.

The motive to write this title was the many photos of typical diseases I have witnessed and then treated during more than 20 years' service at the University of Khartoum Veterinary Clinic (Shambat), during my stay at South Darfur State as a Visiting Assistant Professor, and during field tours with veterinary students to more than 13 states in central, east, and west Sudan between 1985 and 2003 and from visits to Ethiopia, Chad, Kenya, Egypt, the Kingdom of Saudi Arabia, and the Republic of South Africa.

A number of scientific photos have been obtained with courtesy from published or unpublished work of colleagues. Acknowledgments of these sources are provided where relevant. To all who provided such indispensable materials I am very grateful. I appreciate particularly the helpful thoughts of Drs Mohamed Ahmed Hamad, Mohamed Mahmoud Sirdar, Adam Daoud, Mohamed Awad Musa, Kamal Siddig, Hussein Ahmed, Mukhtar T. Abu Samra, Khitma H. Al Malik, Jeruesha Nichols, and Helder Cortes.

A list of references and websites are listed to guide readers to more in-depth knowledge of skin diseases in bovine. Also, the index is complete and contains multiple entries for a single entity when needed.

M.E. Hamid
Current address: College of Medicine, King Khalid University,
Abha, Saudi Arabia

PART I

Clinical Presentations, Laboratory Diagnosis and Disease Summaries

Clinical Quiz No. 1

What is your diagnosis?

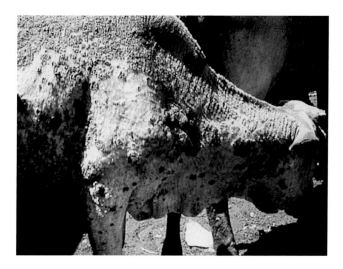

A chronic skin infection in a zebu cow showing exudative dermatitis with heavy scab on the head, neck, and back. Note the enlargement of the superficial lymph nodes. Usually there is little effect on general health of the animal. Early stages show raised clusters of hairs tangled jointly as a wetted paintbrush (typical lesions). When these lesions merge, crusts (scab) are formed which develop to become wart-like lesions ranging from 0.5 to 2 cm in diameter.

LABORATORY DIAGNOSIS

Specimen
- Scabs (crusts, scales)
- Impression smears of the underneath lesions or biopsy.

Skin Diseases of Cattle in the Tropics. DOI: http://dx.doi.org/10.1016/B978-0-12-811054-6.00001-5

Laboratory Tests and Findings

1. Direct detection by microscopic examination (Giemsa or gram stain—see Appendix for details of methods):

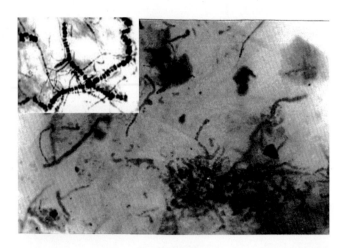

Gram-positive branching filaments with "train track" form or hyphae-like chains.

2. Culture
   a. Fresh uncontaminated scabs or scab emulsions are streaked out directly onto culture media.
   b. Blood agar containing 1000 units/mL of polymyxin B is an effective way to prevent overgrowth by contaminants. Plates are incubated at 37°C under 10% CO_2 for 2−5 days.

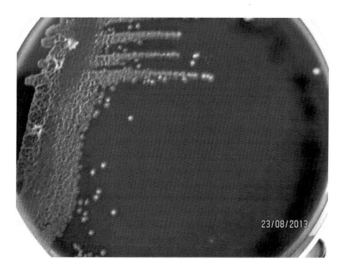

Growth of gray hemolytic colonies that become rough golden with age (Courtesy of doctors: Covarrubias, A.C., Zaragoza, C.S., Bucio, A.M., Aparicio, E.D., Olivares, R.A.C., 2015. CENID Microbiología Instituto Nacional de Investigaciones Forestales Agrícolas y Pecuarias, Mexico).

3. Indirect microscopic examination of grown culture (gram stain):

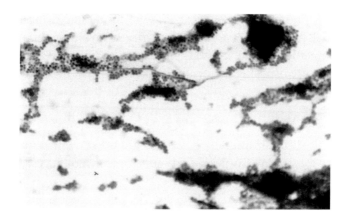

Branching filaments that break up into packets of coccoid cells. Tramcar line-like hyphae can be seen as well.

DIAGNOSIS: DERMATOPHILOSIS (STREPTOTHRICOSIS, RAIN SCALD)

Answer and Disease Summary

Etiology

Dermatophilus congolensis

- A gram-positive facultative anaerobic actinomycete bacterium.
- It has two morphologic forms:
  - Filamentous hyphae (tramcar line-like) and
  - Motile zoospores.
- It grows on sheep-blood enriched agarose media when incubated at 37°C, under a 5–10% CO_2 for 2–4 days as small hemolytic gray-yellow colonies.
- Colonies become rough golden with age to enable isolation of the organism from a contaminated source, antifungal (nystatin) and antibacterial (polymixin) are added to the medium.

Source and Transmission

- *Dermatophilus congolensis* is possibly a soil saprophyte but also the asymptomatic infected animals are regarded as reservoirs.
- It is spread by contact with infected animals, via contaminated environmental objects, and probably via biting insects notably ticks.
- Factors affecting the skin and its integrity such as rain, high humidity, high temperature, and infestation with ticks and lice are considered important predisposing factors in the occurrence of dermatophilosis.

Occurrence

- Worldwide
- Affects all species especially cattle, sheep, horses, and camels
- It is enzootic in tropical and subtropical countries, morbidity 15–100%
- It causes death, loss of hides, fleeces, and is considered a minor zoonotic.

Clinical Findings and Lesions

- An acute or chronic bacterial infection of the epidermis which is characterized by an exudative dermatitis with heavy scab on the back and buttock regions.
- There is evidence of granulomatous surface following shedding of old scabs and enlargement of superficial lymph nodes.

Differential Diagnosis
- Besnoitiosis
- Dermatomycoses in most species
- Warts
- Lumpy skin disease
- Ringworm
- Mange.

Treatment
- Some infected animals may cure without intervention.
- *Dermatophilus congolensis* is sensitive to many antimicrobial agents: amoxicillin, ampicillin, chloramphenicol, erythromycin, gentamycin, novobiocin, penicillin G, spiramycin, streptomycin, and tetracyclines.
- Treatment options:
  - Gently brush the scab and crusts (disinfect infected materials and burn). Then surface is washed or sprayed with:
    - 4% lime sulfur (or hot lime sulfur (97.8% lime sulfur + 2.2% water))
    - 0.5% sodium hypochlorite (1:10 household bleach)
    - 0.5% chlorhexidine
    - 1% povidone-iodine.
  - Systemic application of long-acting oxytetracycline (20 mg/kg) has revealed good results. Also, penicillin + streptomycin or gentamycin are good therapeutic alternatives.

Control and Prevention
- Isolation or culling of infected animals.
- Managing of ectoparasites and sustain skin dry. Particular attention should be given to controlling ticks. Ticks were found to represent a significant risk for the disease development in a number of studies. Tick control may limit the spread of the disease. The use of environmentally safe insecticides sprayed over breeding sites of ticks is recommended. In some countries vector control is not feasible and costly.
- Zinc deficiency and maceration of skin may predispose to infection.

Clinical Quiz No. 2

What is your diagnosis?

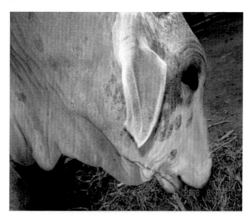

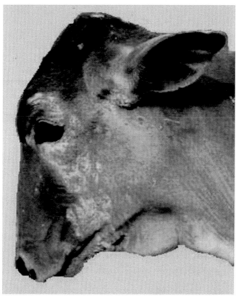

Calves showing painless dermatitis with circular areas of hair loss and thick gray crust which coalesce forming large ash-like surfaces. Crusts were gray-white, oily, and tightly stuck to hair. If detached they cause a red, moist surface that exudes serum or blood.

Skin Diseases of Cattle in the Tropics. DOI: http://dx.doi.org/10.1016/B978-0-12-811054-6.00002-7

LABORATORY DIAGNOSIS

Specimen
- Skin scraping
- Biopsy
- Hair.

Laboratory Tests and Findings

1. Direct microscopy (KOH mount or KOH-Parker ink mount) (see Appendix for details of methods):
   Briefly: In a clean slide place a drop of 10% KOH-Parker ink. Using inoculating needle, place small portion of specimen in the KOH drop, gently heat and wait 20 min. Examine microscopically for faintly blue stained fungal elements.

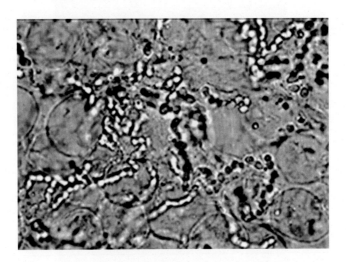

Spores and hyphae breaking up into chains and arthroconidia.

2. Culture on Sabouraud dextrose agar (SDA) (see Appendix for details of methods):
   Place a small portion of infected material (crust, 5–10 hair, or 0.5 mL homogenized material) on the surface of the medium (SDA + Antibiotics). Incubate at 30°C aerobically under high humidity for up to 6 weeks. Examine colony morphology and microscopic features using indirect microscopy.

3. Indirect microscopic examination of grown culture (Lactophenol cotton blue stain or parker ink stain):

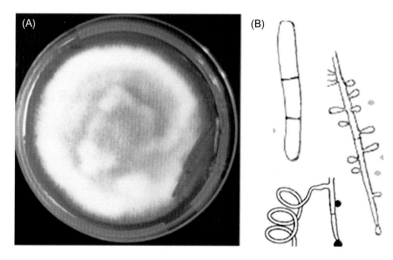

*Growth of gray white to yellow cottony velvety mold colonies (A) and presence of numerous hyaline septate hyphae with macro- and microconidia (*Trichophyton *spp.) (B).*

DIAGNOSIS: DERMATOPHYCOSIS (RINGWORM)

Answer and Disease Summary

Etiology
Dermatophytes

- Dermatophytes are fungi (molds), the etiologic agents of dermatophytoses or ringworm
- They are classified in three anamorphic (asexual or imperfect) genera:
  - *Epidermophyton*
  - *Microsporum*
  - *Trichophyton.*
- They cause skin, hair, and nail infections.

Source and Transmission
- Spores of dermatophytes are able to persist for years in environment including hot dry weather.
- Infections spread via the direct contact with infected animals.

Occurrence
- Worldwide
- All species are affected especially cattle, sheep, horses, and camels
- It is enzootic in tropical and subtropical countries
- It causes loss of hides, fleeces, and is considered a minor zoonotic.

Clinical Findings and Lesions
- An acute or chronic fungal infection of epidermis
- It is characterized by dermatitis with scab on the face, neck, and back.

Differential Diagnosis
- Mange
- Dermatophilosis
- Besnoitasis
- Also, differentiate it from conditions with hyperkeratosis, parakeratosis, pityriasis, and pachyderma.

Treatment
- Infected cattle mostly recover spontaneously.
- Treatment options for valuable animals:
  - Gently brush the scab and crusts, and then disinfect infected materials and burn.

- Treatment options include wash or sprays with:
  - 4% lime sulfur (or hot lime sulfur (97.8% lime sulfur + 2.2% water)).
  - 0.5% sodium hypochlorite (1:10 household bleach)
  - 0.5% chlorhexidine
  - 1% povidone-iodine
  - Antifungal lotions.
- Lesions can be treated with antifungals: miconazole or clotrimazole lotions.
- Usually animals recover in about 10 days after treatment.

Control and Prevention
- Effective control of ringworm requires proper cleaning and disinfecting of animal locations and equipment. A strong disinfectant such as hypochlorite (1:10 household bleach) is an excellent choice which helps to avoid infecting healthy animals.
- Scab and crusts removed before treatment, have to be disinfected and destroyed.
- A live attenuated fungal vaccine is available in the United States.

Clinical Quiz No. 3

What is your diagnosis?

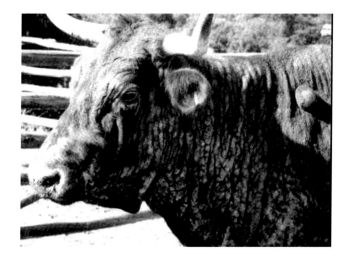

A cow showing chronic skin lesion with exudative dermatitis, advancing thickening, folding, or wrinkling of the skin with hair loss, cracks, scabs, edema, and enlargement of superficial lymph nodes. Mucopurulent nasal discharge and lameness due to sole ulcers may be noticed. In acute stage, there is pyrexia, serous nasal and ocular discharges, inappetence with weight loss, photophobia, reluctance to move, and skin hyperemia. Photo courtesy of Dr. Helder Cortes: Laboratório de Parasitologia, ICAM, Universidade de E´vora, Portugal.

LABORATORY DIAGNOSIS

Specimen
- Skin biopsy from infected tissue.

Skin Diseases of Cattle in the Tropics. DOI: http://dx.doi.org/10.1016/B978-0-12-811054-6.00003-9

Laboratory Tests and Findings

1. Histopathological examination (H&E) (see Appendix for details of methods):

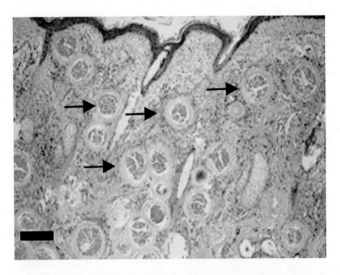

Histopathology (paraffin section) of a skin lesion of a cow showing intradermal cysts (arrows) containing hundreds of parasites (bradizoytes), associated with inflammatory cell infiltrates (Bar = 200 mm, H&E). Courtesy of Dr. Helder Cortes: Laboratório de Parasitologia, ICAM, Universidade de É´vora, Portugal.

DIAGNOSIS: BOVINE BESNOITIOSIS (ELEPHANT SKIN DISEASE)

Answer and Disease Summary

Etiology

Besnoitia besnoiti

- *Besnoitia besnoiti* is an obligate intracellular protozoan parasite belonging to the phylum apicomplexan.
- It is similar to *Toxoplasma.*
- It multiplies in macrophages and endothelial and other cells, producing large, thick-walled cysts filled with bradyzoites.
- The cysts grow to become invading tachyzoites.
- Stinging insects such as tabanid and stomoxy are thought to play a role in the transmission of this disease.

Source and Transmission

- Horizontal transmission following direct contact between animals with wounds or lacerations where cysts can be found is one of the methods of spread.
- Infected bulls during mating have been suggested.
- Biting flies, for instance, horseflies and deerflies, are thought to act as mechanical transmitters of the infection.
- But the exact routes of transmission and risk factors of infection with *B. besnoiti* remain unknown.

Occurrence

- Possibly worldwide.
- It affects cattle (over 6 month old), horses and donkeys, and occasionally goats.
- The disease is spread by biting flies but infection may also come from cats, which are assumed as the final host of *Besnoitia besnoiti.*
- Cats are known to excrete *Besnoitia* oocysts in their feces.

Clinical Findings and Lesions

- Affected animals may have high fever, photophobia (avoidance of direct sunlight), edema of the skin, diarrhea, and enlargement of superficial lymph nodes.
- Up to 10% of affected animals die in the early stage.
- Survivors develop a chronic disease in which the parasites localize in cysts underneath the skin.
- Marked scleroderma in legs, dorsum, and nose.

Differential Diagnosis
- Febrile stage can be confused with acute diseases such as:
  - Heartwater
  - Red water
  - Acute photosensitization
  - Malignant catarrhal fever
- The skin lesions and scleroderma stage are similar to:
  - Dermatophilosis
  - Mange
  - Lumpy skin disease
  - Poisoning with mercury and chlorinated naphthalenes.

Treatment
- Treatment is difficult and of limited success.
- Wound dressing, control of secondary infections, control of insect, and providing shade and nutrition for sick animals are good supportive treatments.
- Oxytetracycline (long acting; 20 mg/kg, repeated 2 days later) during the initial stages showed good results. Similar results by using antimony and sulfanilamide.

Control and Prevention
- Separating sick animals from healthy ones or culling have shown to decrease the appearance of new cases.
- An effective vaccine is available in South Africa.

Clinical Quiz No. 4

What is your diagnosis?

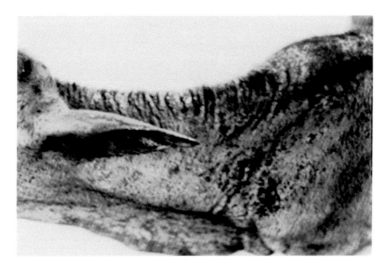

A calf showing dermatitis with areas of hair loss, folds, and thin to thick scab on the head, neck, perineum, dewlap, and extending to other parts of the body. It is characterized by intense pruritus, hair loss, papules that progress to scabs and crusts, and skin thickens to massive folds.

LABORATORY DIAGNOSIS

Specimen
- Skin scraping
- Biopsy.

Skin Diseases of Cattle in the Tropics. DOI: http://dx.doi.org/10.1016/B978-0-12-811054-6.00004-0

Laboratory Tests and Findings

1. Direct microscopy (10% KOH mount) (see Appendix for details of methods):

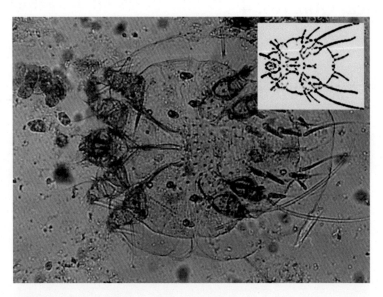

A spherical arthropod parasite with four pairs of legs seen in skin scraping of a cow suffering from dermatitis that is characterized by areas of hair loss, folds, and thin to thick scab.

DIAGNOSIS: SARCOPTIC MANGE (SCABIES)

Answer and Disease Summary

Etiology

Sarcoptes scabiei (mites)

- *Sarcoptes scabiei* or the itch mite is a parasitic arthropod that burrows into skin and causes scabies.
- Adult scabies mites are spherical, eyeless mites with four pairs of legs.
- They are recognizable by their oval, ventrally flattened and dorsally convex tortoise-like body and multiple cuticular.

Source and Transmission

- Under farm conditions, mites do not survive outside animal host for long (c. 3 days).
- Spread occurs mainly via direct contact between infected and noninfected animals.
- Transmission also occurs through contacts with contaminated environmental materials or fomites.

Occurrence

- Worldwide
- All species especially cattle, sheep, horses, and camels
- It is enzootic in tropical and subtropical countries
- It causes loss of hides, fleeces, and it is regarded as a minor zoonotic.

Clinical Findings and Lesions

- Dermatitis on the head, neck, and perineum
- It is characterized by hair loss, skin folds, and thin to thick scab.

Differential diagnosis

- Dermatophilosis
- Demodectic mange
- Dermatophytosis
- Zinc deficiency
- Besnoitiosis.

Treatment
- Application of insecticides by spray, dipping, oral, topical, or injectable formulations of systemic drugs, such as macrocyclic lactones or organophosphate insecticides or lime sulfur, is effective:
  - A number of macrocyclic lactone compounds are available for use in animals and include avermectin, abamectin, doramectin, eprinomectin, milbemycins, moxidectin, and selamectin.
    - The efficacy of ivermectin long-acting injection formulation was very successful.
  - Organophosphates used topically, which include coumaphos, diazinon, dichlorvos, famphur, fenthion, malathion, trichlorfon, stirofos, phosmet, and propetamphos.
  - Pyrethroids: Some of the more common pyrethroids used include bioallethrin, cypermethrin, deltamethrin, fenvalerate, flumethrin, lambdacyhalothrin, phenothrin, and permethrin. Animals should be wet thoroughly with the product and retreated in 10 − 14 days. Permethrin cream or lotion is available for topical use.
  - Hot lime sulfur (97.8% lime sulfur + 2.2% water or inert ingredient) used as dips or sprays and repeated at 12-day intervals for two to three times is effective for general nonspecific skin conditions (avoid contact with eyes and mucous membranes).

Control and Prevention
- Clean contaminated places and equipment by spraying of insecticides to avoid infecting healthy animals. Many formulations of insecticides are available commercially.
- Isolate affected animals from susceptible ones (long incubation period represents a sound difficulty).

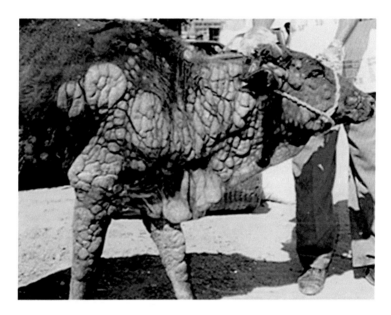

Clinical Quiz No. 5

What is your diagnosis?

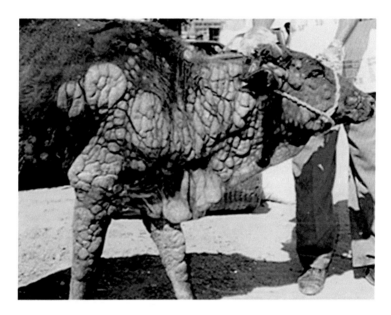

Dermatitis with massive thick, scaly, and nodular folds mainly covering the head, neck, and shoulders on a 2-year-old Friesian–Kenana cross-breed cow. It is characterized by pruritus, hair loss, papules that progress to scabs and crusts, and very thick folds.

LABORATORY DIAGNOSIS

Specimen
- Skin scraping
- Biopsy.

Skin Diseases of Cattle in the Tropics. DOI: http://dx.doi.org/10.1016/B978-0-12-811054-6.00005-2

Laboratory Tests and Findings

1. Direct microscopy: (10% KOH mount; or H&E):

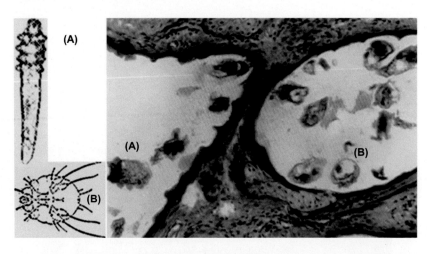

Presence of both elongated arthropod parasite with four pairs of legs (A) and spherical-body parasites (B) seen in an H&E stained skin section of a heifer with massive cutaneous lesions.

DIAGNOSIS: SARCOPTIC AND DEMODECTIC MANGE (MIXED MANGE)

Answer and Disease Summary

Etiology

- *Sarcoptes scabiei* (Sarcoptic)
- *Demodex bovis* (Demodectic).

Source and Transmission

- As for sarcoptic and demodectic mange, mites do not survive outside animal host for long (c. 3 days).
- Spread occurs mainly via direct contact between infected and noninfected animals.
- Transmission also occurs through contact with contaminated environmental materials or fomites.

Occurrence

- Rare, mainly cattle.

Clinical Findings and Lesions

- Lumps of granulomatous tumor-like dermatitis
- With thick, nodular folds
- Mainly covering the head, neck, and shoulders.

Differential Diagnosis

- Besnoitasis
- Dermatophilosis
- Warts.

Treatment

- Treatment is difficult in such advanced cases.
- Early stages are treatable with application of:
  - A number of macrocyclic lactone compounds are available for use in animals and include avermectins, abamectin, doramectin, eprinomectin, ivermectin, milbemycins, moxidectin, and selamectin
    - The efficacy of ivermectin long-acting injection formulation was very successful.
  - Organophosphates used topically which include coumaphos, diazinon, dichlorvos, famphur, fenthion, malathion, trichlorfon, stirofos, phosmet, and propetamphos.
  - Pyrethroids: Some of the more common pyrethroids used include bioallethrin, cypermethrin, deltamethrin, fenvalerate, flumethrin,

lambdacyhalothrin, phenothrin, and permethrin. Animals should be wet thoroughly with the product and retreated after $10-14$ days. Permethrin cream or lotion is available for topical use.

- Hot lime sulfur (97.8% lime sulfur + 2.2% water or inert ingredient) used as dips or sprays and repeated at 12-day intervals for two to three times is effective for general nonspecific skin conditions (avoid contact with eyes and mucous membranes).
- Heavy scab and crusts may require gentle removal and then surface is washed or sprayed with 4% lime sulfur (or hot lime sulfur (97.8% lime sulfur + 2.2% water)), or 0.5% sodium hypochlorite (1:10 household bleach) or 0.5% chlorhexidine or 1% povidone-iodine. This adjuvant treatment goes along with the above insecticidal therapy.

Control and Prevention
- Control similar to other types of mange:
  - Clean contaminated places and equipment by the spraying insecticides to avoid infecting healthy animals. Many formulations of insecticides are available commercially.
  - Isolate affected animals from susceptible ones (long incubation period represents a sound difficulty).

Clinical Quiz No. 6

What is your diagnosis?

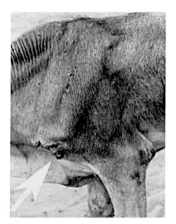

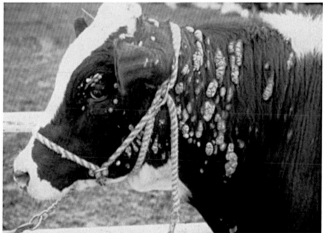

Skin lesions on prescapular area of a zebu calf (top) and on the head and neck of a Friesian cow (below). Lesions are tumor-like in appearance; they stay for a prolonged time and appear as unconnected low flat and circular shapes which may become characteristically pendulous. Source: Lower photo courtesy of Dr. Jeruesha Nichols, CVT Colorado State University.

Skin Diseases of Cattle in the Tropics. DOI: http://dx.doi.org/10.1016/B978-0-12-811054-6.00006-4

LABORATORY DIAGNOSIS

Specimen
- Biopsy of infected tissues
- Blood.

Laboratory Tests and Findings
1. Blood/serum
   a. ELISA
2. Biopsy, infected tissues
   a. Molecular diagnosis
      Amplification and sequencing of the L1 gene
   b. Electron microscopy

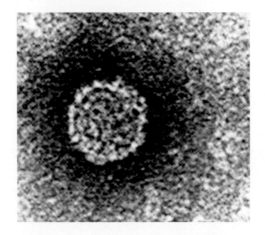

Hexagonal shape of wart virus particles seen in purified suspension of wart-infected tissue. Source: Swain and Dodds, 1967, Clinical Virology, Edinburgh: Churchill Livingstone.

DIAGNOSIS: PAPILLOMATOSIS (WARTS)

Answer and Disease Summary

Etiology

Bovine papillomaviruses (BPV)

- BPV is a group of DNA virus of the family *Papillomaviridae*
- The virus infects particularly body surface of cattle.

Source and Transmission

- Papillomatosis spreads by direct or indirect contact
- Organism enters animal through skin abrasions
- Papillomavirus DNA has been detected in blood, milk, urine, and other body fluids of infected animals.

Occurrence

- Worldwide
- Found generally in mammals and birds as cutaneous and mucosal tumors
- Very common in younger animals (under 2 years) and generally spontaneously regresses
- Cattle and horses, worldwide
- Morbidity 20%, case fatality 2%
- The virus is resistant to extreme cold and heat
- That is why it is not uncommon to find cattle with warts during all seasons and in all types of cattle.

Clinical Findings and Lesions

- Incubation period 3–8 weeks
- It starts with solid outgrowths of skin and connective tissue
- On any part of the body
- Lesions pedunculated smooth or ulcerative cauliflower in appearance
- It causes loss of milk, weight, and hides.

Differential Diagnosis

- Besnoitasis
- Dermatophilosis
- Ringworm.

Treatment

- Warts are generally not serious
- Usually disappear spontaneously and lesions fall off or shrink after about 6 months

- Warts can be crushed (removed) at their early stages
- Removal of warts surgically—thought intolerable—but can be a treatment choice. Dressing of wound is necessary and control of secondary infections.

Control and Prevention
- Isolate affected animals from susceptible ones (long incubation period represents a sound difficulty)
- A commercial wart vaccine is available (Colorado Serum Company). It stimulates immunity by increasing the amount of virus in the bloodstream postvaccination. A booster dose is given 3−5 weeks later.

Clinical Quiz No. 7

What is your diagnosis?

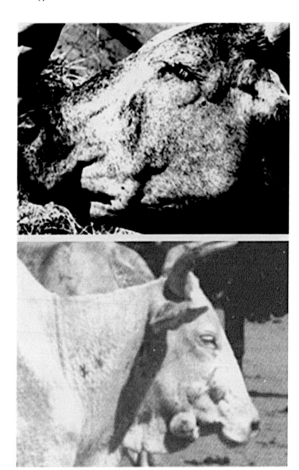

Chronic, localized bony swellings on the mandible, maxilla, and surrounding tissues of adult cows. Lesions are characterized by painless, immovable progressive, granulomatous abscesses which affect the skin and nearby bones. Infections may result in facial deformation, loss of teeth, and dyspnea as a result of nasal obstruction. Ulcers with fistulas with exudate drainage can appear.

Skin Diseases of Cattle in the Tropics. DOI: http://dx.doi.org/10.1016/B978-0-12-811054-6.00007-6

LABORATORY DIAGNOSIS

Specimen
- Biopsy
- Discharges and grains
- Aspirate.

Laboratory Tests and Findings
1. Direct microscopy: (H&E)

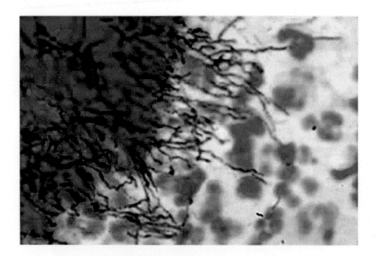

Branching gram-positive filaments on the edge of granules (sulfur granules). Source: Harriet Provine, Boston, MA.

2. Culture (blood agar/anaerobic/37°C/2–4 days)

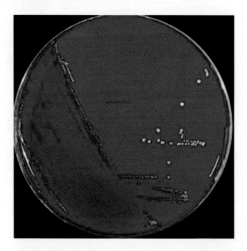

Small smooth convex colonies on blood agar. Anaerobic culture at 37°C, 2–4 days. Source: www.vetbact.se.

3. Indirect microscopic examination of grown culture (gram stain)

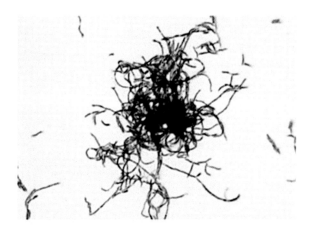

Gram-positive branching filamentous of Actinomyces bovis. Source: www.studyblue.com.

DIAGNOSIS: ACTINOMYCOSIS (LUMPY JAW)

Answer and Disease Summary

Etiology

Actinomyces bovis

- *Actinomyces bovis* is a gram-positive, facultative anaerobic, nonspore forming bacterium in the genus *Actinomyces* of the class Actinobacteria.
- It grows best under anaerobic conditions.
- Microscopically, it forms fungus-like branched networks of hyphae.

Source and Transmission

- Pathogenic *Actinomyces* spp. do not survive outside host tissue.
- They are normal flora of the nasopharyngeal gastrointestinal tract, and female genital tract. *Actinomyces* spp. gain access to subcutaneous soft tissue through wounds of the oral mucosa caused by sharp objects, such as wire or rough grass or sticks.
- Wounds in the oral mucosae initiated by sharp objects, such as wires, hay, chewing and eating abrasive feed or sharp branches, are obvious risk factors.

Occurrence

- Widespread
- A minor zoonotic
- It is common only in cattle, rare in pigs.

Clinical Findings and Lesions

- A localized granulomatous infection
- Characterized by the formation of painless immovable, bony swellings on the mandible, maxilla, and surrounding tissues
- The lesions enlarge over time
- Sinuses discharge sticky yellow-white pus which may contain grains.

Differential Diagnosis

- Abscesses
- Foreign bodies
- Bovine farcy
- Skin tuberculosis (tuberculous lymphadenitis)
- Chronic lesions of lumpy skin disease
- Wooden tongue (actinobacillosis).

Treatment
- No effective treatment is available.
- Treatment during the initial stages of the disease with penicillin, sulfonamides, or cephalosporins is generally positive as the causative agent is sensitive to many antimicrobial agents.
- Abscess draining and wound caring is needed. When the infection penetrates bones, treatment requires meticulous work to be successful.
- Surgical cauterization or removal and debridement could be useful.

Control and Prevention
- Isolate or cull (sent to an abattoir for slaughter) affected animals.
- In case of large discharging abscess, affected animals should be destroyed and affected animals premises should be disinfected. A strong disinfectant such as hypochlorite (1:10 household bleach) is a good choice.
- Check for new cases, then isolate to decrease environmental contamination.
- Manage grazing to decrease exposure of cattle to coarse or prickly feed.

Clinical Quiz No. 8

What is your diagnosis?

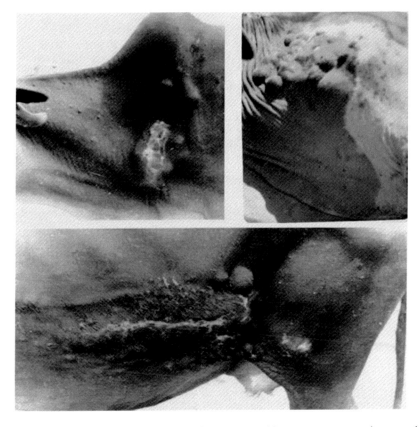

Zebu cows showing lymphocutaneous clusters of hard up to 10 cm nodules. Lesions are seen on the prescapular and femoral regions, gradually progressing and enlarging, coalescing and may open to exterior discharging pus. Characteristically, lesions may appear cord-like along the lymphatic vessels.

LABORATORY DIAGNOSIS

Specimen
- Biopsy

Skin Diseases of Cattle in the Tropics. DOI: http://dx.doi.org/10.1016/B978-0-12-811054-6.00008-8

- Discharge
- Aspirate.

Laboratory Tests and Findings

1. Direct microscopy: Ziehl Neelsen stain (see Appendix for details of methods)

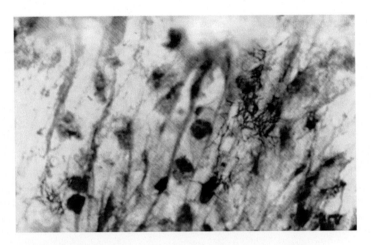

Acid-fast branching filamentous organisms. Filaments are arranged in clumps or tangled lacy network which do not fragment into bacillary forms and are strongly acid-alcohol fast.

2. Culture (Lowenstein Jensen/aerobic/37°C/1−3 weeks)

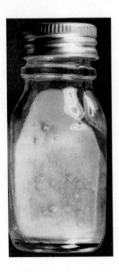

Growth of nonchromogenic, wheat-colored, cream yellow rough, raised wrinkled colonies.

DIAGNOSIS: BOVINE FARCY (NOCARDIOSIS)

Answer and Disease Summary

Etiology

Mycobacterium species

- *Mycobacterium farcinogenes* (East and Central Africa) and *Mycobacterium senegalense* (West Africa).
- These actinomycetes are closely related to *Nocardia farcinica* (previously considered the cause of this disease).
- *M. farcinogenes* and *M. senegalense* are aerobic, gram-positive, acid-fast, short or long branching filaments that are arranged in clumps or tangled lacy network.
- The growth on Lowenstein Jensen medium is slow and colonies appear as nonchromogenic, wheat-colored, rough convoluted, and irregular.

Source and Transmission

- The route of infection is unknown, organism may enter through abrasions and wounds caused by thorns of shrubs.
- Soil contaminated by discharge and ticks are possible sources of infection.
- There are no reports of isolations or detections of *M. farcinogenes* and *M. senegalense* in environmental samples.

Occurrence

- Found in Africa
- Mainly in adults cattle of the transhumance pastoralist tribes of the Sahel and the Sudanian savannah zones.

Clinical Findings and Lesions

- A chronic infectious disease of cattle characterized by lympho-cutaneous granulomatous inflammations.
- Slowly progressive, small to large hard subcutaneous nodules are formed.
- Common at the prescapular, precrural, and parotid regions to generalized.
- Lesions rupture, discharging thick gray or yellow granular or cheesy pus.
- Lesions may heal spontaneously.

Differential Diagnosis
- Abscesses
- Foreign bodies
- Actinomycosis
- Skin tuberculosis (tuberculous lymphadentitis)
- Chronic lesions of lumpy skin disease.

Treatment
- Effective treatment is not available.
- Most of the *M. farcinogenes* and *M. senegalense* strains tested *in vitro* were found susceptible to cycloserine, dapsone, amikacin, doxycycline HCl, oxytetracycline HCl, and paromomycin sulfate (64 μg/mL).
- Long-term therapy (1−6 months) is required but seems not practical under field conditions especially under nomadic situations.
- Surgical procedures with focus on debridement, drainage, and washing of lesions with antiseptic solutions such as 0.5% chlorhexidine or 1% iodine may be useful.
- Cauterization is practice by some tribes.

Control and Prevention
- Specific preventive and effective measures to control bovine farcy are not available. This could be due to the fact that bovine farcy and nocardiosis have wide distribution in the environment and that transmission and risk factors are not fully understood.
- Tick control may limit the spread of the disease as for dermatophilosis. The use of environmentally safe insecticides sprayed over breeding sites of ticks is recommended. In some countries vector control is not feasible and costly.

Clinical Quiz No. 9

What is your diagnosis?

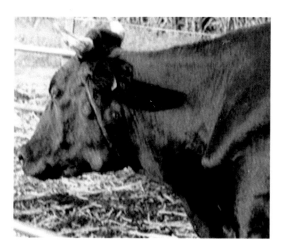

A cow (Friesian−Kenana cross) showing chronic small to large hard subcutaneous nodules. Lesions are seen at the prescapular, precrural, and parotid lymph nodes and could be generalized. Lesions develop in size and gradually spread, frequently ulcerating releasing thick pus.

LABORATORY DIAGNOSIS

Specimen
- Biopsy
- Discharge
- Aspirate.

Skin Diseases of Cattle in the Tropics. DOI: http://dx.doi.org/10.1016/B978-0-12-811054-6.00009-X

Laboratory Tests and Findings
1. Direct microscopy: Ziehl Neelsen stain

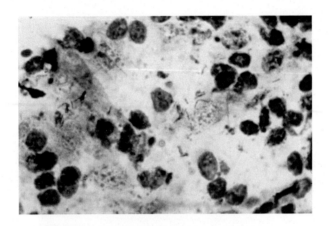

Acid-fast bacilli (red) on a blue background, characteristic for Mycobacterium *spp.*

2. Culture (Lowenstein Jensen/aerobic/37°C/2−6 weeks)

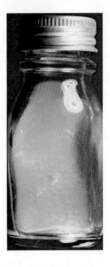

Growth of cream yellow, rough colonies on Lowenstein Jensen medium.

DIAGNOSIS: SKIN TUBERCULOSIS (TUBERCULOUS LYMPHADENITIS)

Answer and Disease Summary

Etiology
- *Mycobacterium avium*
- Also, *Mycobacterium kansasii, Mycobacterium intracellulare, Mycobacterium fortuitum* are sometimes implicated
- These mycobacteria are slow-growing aerobic, gram-positive, acid-fast bacteria.

Source and Transmission
- Mycobacteria other than *Mycobacterium tuberculosis* and *Mycobacterium leprae* usually survive outside human or animal hosts as free living saprophytes in the environment.
- Domestic animals as well as wildlife are significant reservoir hosts for human tuberculosis, caused by *Mycobacterium bovis*. Sustained contact with soil has also been recognized as one of the risk factors.
- Infections may occur as a result of exposure to contaminated environments via abrasion, laceration, or bite wounds.

Occurrence
- Uncommon
- But some cases among housed cattle are encountered.

Clinical Findings and Lesions
- Slowly progressive, small to large hard subcutaneous nodules seen mostly at the prescapular, precrural, and parotid lymph nodes or generalized
- Open to exterior discharging pus
- It sensitizes cattle to tuberculin skin testing.

Differential Diagnosis
- Bovine farcy
- Abscesses
- Actinomycosis
- Chronic lesions of lumpy skin disease.

Treatment
- Effective treatment is not available.
- Long-term therapy (1−6 months) is required, especially in high valued cattle such as the Friesian and cross-breeds. This usually

involves a combination of antibiotics (isoniazid, rifampicin, pyrazinamide, and ethambutol) given over a period of several months.
- Surgical procedures with focus on debridement, drainage, and washing of lesions with antiseptic solutions such as 0.5% chlorhexidine or 1% iodine may be useful.
- Cauterization is practiced by some.

Control and Prevention
- Similar to bovine tuberculosis and bovine farcy there are no specifically known measures to control this mycobacteriosis.
- Confirmed positive mycobacteriosis cases should be isolated or culled.
- Affected animals with discharging abscess should be destroyed and affected animals' premises should be disinfected. A strong disinfectant such as hypochlorite (1:10 household bleach) is a good choice.

Clinical Quiz No. 10

What is your diagnosis?

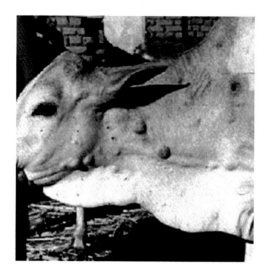

A calf showing chronic multiple round intradermal painless hard nodules (1–4 cm). Lesions may harden and persist for a long time or may slough out leaving holes on the skin (sitfast or saddle sore). Severe skin inflammation caused by secondary infection of the lesions devastates the animal's condition.

LABORATORY DIAGNOSIS

Specimen
- Tissue and blood samples.

Laboratory Tests and Findings
1. Blood (serum)
   a. Serological tests
   b. FA (fluorescent antibody)

Skin Diseases of Cattle in the Tropics. DOI: http://dx.doi.org/10.1016/B978-0-12-811054-6.00010-6

    c. Virus neutralization

    d. ELISA for antigen-detection (sample should be taken during the first week of signs, before neutralizing antibodies develop)

2. EDTA blood, semen, biopsy, or tissue culture samples

    a. Molecular analysis

    Highly sensitive and specific. Strains are identified by sequence and phylogenetic analysis

3. Tissue

    a. Histopathological examination (H&E)

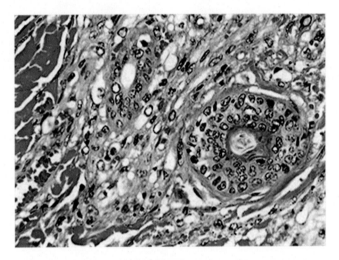

Perifollicular histiocytic inflammation. Note histiocyte-like cells with large vacuolated nuclei and eosinophilic intranuclear inclusions (H&E). Source: Foreign Animal Disease Diagnostic Lab, USDA-APHIS.

DIAGNOSIS: LUMPY SKIN DISEASE (CHRONIC LESIONS)

Answer and Disease Summary

Etiology

Neethling poxvirus (*Poxviridae*)

- Serotype: Lumpy Skin Disease Virus (LSDV); Family: *Poxviridae*; Genus: *Capripoxvirus* (also Sheep Pox and Goat Pox).
- Can be recovered from skin nodules kept at $-80°C$ for 10 years and infected tissue culture fluid stored at $4°C$ for 6 months.
- Survives for long periods at ambient temperature especially in dried scabs.

Source and Transmission

- Sources for transmission of lumpy skin disease are cutaneous lesions and crusts.
- Virus is also present in blood, nasal secretions, secretions, milk, semen, and saliva.
- Factors such as the agro-climates, communal grazing/watering management, and introduction of new animals were significantly associated with the occurrence of lumpy skin disease.
- Also, an increase in the biting-fly population is regarded as a transmission factor.

Occurrence

- Enzootic in Africa
- A disease of cattle
- Morbidity 20%, case fatality 2%
- Cause loss of milk, weight, and hides.

Clinical Findings and Lesions

- Skin lesions appear after 1 week of fever, lacrimation, and nasal discharge.
- Lesions are multiple and about 1–4 cm intradermal nodules.
- Lesions usually recover in 2–4 weeks, some persist for years.

Differential Diagnosis

- Pseudo-lumpy skin disease
- Urticarial
- Bovine ulcerative mammillitis
- Bovine farcy
- Abscesses.

Treatment
- No specific treatment is available.
- The chronic lesions are harmless with some effect on the quality of skin.
- Strong antibiotic therapy prevents secondary infection, eg, long-acting oxytetracycline (20 mg/kg).

Control and Prevention
- Virus spreads rapidly, therefore restriction of animal movement and quarantine restrictions are of limited use.
- Homologous live attenuated vaccine is available, immunity lasts up to 3 years.

Clinical Quiz No. 11

What is your diagnosis?

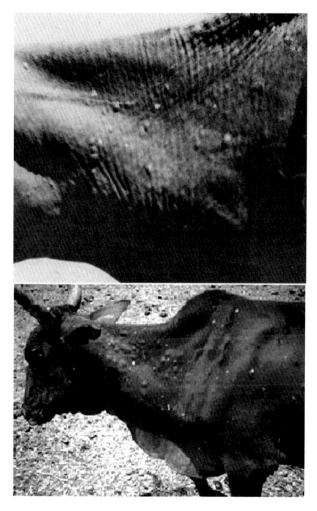

Cows with skin lesions showing rough, folded skins with many small (top cow) and large (bottom cow) soft to hard abscesses (folliculitis) releasing purulent cheesy materials upon pressure.

Skin Diseases of Cattle in the Tropics. DOI: http://dx.doi.org/10.1016/B978-0-12-811054-6.00011-8

LABORATORY DIAGNOSIS

Specimen
- Biopsy (tissue section)
- Pus and discharge.

Laboratory Tests and Findings
1. Direct microscopy (KOH mount)

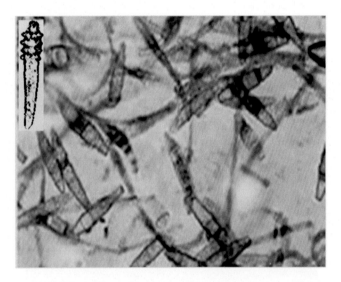

Cigar-shaped elongated arthropod parasites with four pairs of short legs seen in a 10% KOH mount made from pus of nodular skin lesions in a zebu cow.

DIAGNOSIS: DEMODECTIC MANGE (DEMODICOSIS)

Answer and Disease Summary

Etiology
Demodex bovis

- *Demodex* is a genus of mite in the family *Demodicidae*. Demodectic or follicular mite is an elongated mite about 0.25 mm long with four pairs of stout short legs and a long abdomen transversely striated on top and bottom.
- Life cycle thought to be similar to other mites.
- Mites enter hair follicles and sebaceous glands of the skin, causing chronic inflammation, thickening of skin, and hair loss.
- Bacteria, frequently staphylococci, enter and kindle abscess and nodule formation.

Source and Transmission
- The life cycle of *Demodex* mite (ova, larvae, nymphs, and adults) is about 10−15 days and takes place in the epidermis.
- Mites and ova survive away from the host for only short periods of time.
- Depending on temperature and humidity, mites may survive for up to 15 days outside the dermis.

Occurrence
- The disease is mainly found in tropical countries.
- Dogs and cattle are the most affected species.

Clinical Findings and Lesions
- Lesions on brisket, lower neck, shoulder, forearm, and back.
- Lesions are not readily visible (detected on hides as holes).
- On palpation, pustules which contain white cheesy pus can be touched.
- No irritation but skin thickened and hair loss in some areas.

Differential Diagnosis
- Urticaria
- Deep ringworm
- Staphylococcal dermatitis
- Filarial dermatitis
- Sporotrichosis.

Treatment
- Treatment is difficult.
- Application of systemic ivermectin or organophosphorus compounds might be of value.
  - Avermectins and Milbemycins: avermectins abamectin, doramectin, eprinomectin, ivermectin, milbemycins, moxidectin, and selamectin.
    - Ivermectin is the most commonly used and available.
  - Organophosphate insecticides:
    - Organophosphates used topically include coumaphos, diazinon, dichlorvos, famphur, fenthion, malathion, trichlorfon, stirofos, phosmet, and propetamphos.
- Antibiotic application to severely damage areas prevents secondary infections, eg, long-acting oxytetracycline (20 mg/kg).

Control and Prevention
- Control similar to other types of mange:
  - Clean contaminated places and equipment by the spraying of insecticides to avoid infecting healthy animals. Many formulations of insecticides are available commercially.
  - Isolate affected animals from susceptible ones (long incubation period represents a sound difficulty).

Clinical Quiz No. 12

What is your diagnosis?

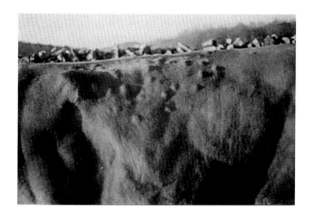

A cow showing soft nodular swellings on the subcutis. Aspirate reveals no purulent or watery materials. Larvae embedded in skin can be seen over each swelling which displays holes. Larvae then rest with the posterior stigmal plate pointed towards the pore to breathe. Source: http://www.vetnext.com/1987.

LABORATORY DIAGNOSIS

Specimen
- Infected tissue biopsy.

Laboratory Tests and Findings
1. Visual examination
   a. Check the presence of flies of the genus *Hypoderma*, order *Diptera* in animal's environment.

Skin Diseases of Cattle in the Tropics. DOI: http://dx.doi.org/10.1016/B978-0-12-811054-6.00012-X

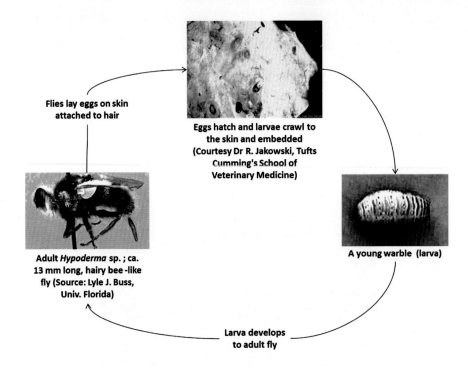

Flies lay eggs on skin attached to hair

Eggs hatch and larvae crawl to the skin and embedded (Courtesy Dr R. Jakowski, Tufts Cumming's School of Veterinary Medicine)

Adult *Hypoderma* sp. ; ca. 13 mm long, hairy bee -like fly (Source: Lyle J. Buss, Univ. Florida)

A young warble (larva)

Larva develops to adult fly

DIAGNOSIS: CUTANEOUS HYPODERMATITIS (CATTLE GRUBS)

Answer and Disease Summary

Etiology
- Larvae of flies of *Hypoderma* spp. (Warble fly) and *Dermatobia hominis*.
- Adult warble flies are parasites of cattle and deer.
- They are large hairy and bee-like; brown, orange, or yellow in color.

Source and Transmission
- The cattle grub lives in regions where there are plentiful host animals.
- The fly lays eggs on the foreleg of the affected cattle.
- These will be ingested by licking, and be swallowed. Internal cycle involves passing through the esophagus muscles and spinal cord and then emerging subcutaneously.
- Life cycle usually extends for a year.

Occurrence
- Worldwide
- Mainly cattle.

Clinical Findings and Lesions
- Soft nodular swelling on the subcutis
- Larvae embedded in skin
- Various inflammation and may be necrosis in skin and tissues.

Differential Diagnosis
- Demodectic mange
- Filarial dermatitis
- Sporotrichosis
- Skin lesions of lumpy skin disease.

Treatment
- Mature cattle grubs can be squeezed out of the warble through the breathing hole:
  Pour-on and spot-on application of insecticide is effective.
- Systemic insecticides are more effective. Examples: ivermectin or organophosphorus insecticides in various formulations are effective:
  Avermectins and Milbemycins: avermectins, abamectin, doramectin, eprinomectin, ivermectin, milbemycins, moxidectin, and selamectin.
  Ivermectin is the most commonly used and widely available.

Organophosphate insecticides: Organophosphates used topically include coumaphos, diazinon, dichlorvos, famphur, fenthion, malathion, trichlorfon, stirofos, phosmet, and propetamphos.
- Dressing of wounds: debridement, drainage, removal of foreign bodies, and washing of lesions with antiseptic solutions.
- Antibiotic application to severely damaged areas prevents secondary infections, eg, long-acting oxytetracycline (20 mg/kg).

Control and Prevention
- Larvae control: larvae can be controlled by applying or dusting insecticides, such as tetrachlorvinphos, to the warbles in the back. Treatment must be repeated every 30–45 days during the warble season to control newly appearing grubs.
- Fly control: spraying insecticides to animal premises to avoid infecting healthy animals. Some environmentally friendly formulations of insecticides are available commercially.

Clinical Quiz No. 13

What is your diagnosis?

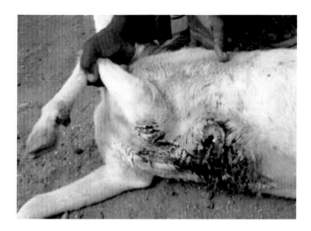

A calf showing massive wounds on the ventral thorax and abdomen. The wounds were caused by attacks by flies which lay eggs causing irritation, large, soft, painful swellings; then swellings ulcerate causing damage to hide and flesh. Symptoms include itching and perception of pain and annoyance. In early lesions the presence of a central opening with serosanguinous drainage distinguishes these lesions from bacterial furunculosis and arthropod bites. Source: Photo courtesy of The Yemeni Ministry of Agriculture's General Department for Animal Resources (GDAR), Sanaa.

LABORATORY DIAGNOSIS

Specimen
- Collect maggots embedded in cutaneous tissue.

Laboratory Tests and Findings
1. Examine lesions
2. Examine lesions: soft to hard abscess with purulent materials and ulcers

Skin Diseases of Cattle in the Tropics. DOI: http://dx.doi.org/10.1016/B978-0-12-811054-6.00013-1

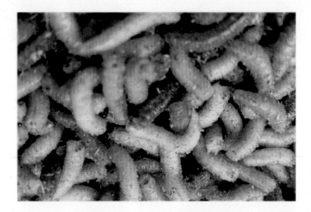

Maggots embedded in cutaneous tissues

Check flies: Check presence of flies in animal environment.

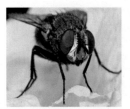

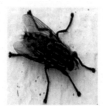

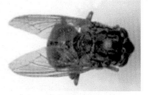

Blow fly (*Calliphoridae*)
(Phot courtesy Martin Pot
http://martybugs.net/blog)

Flesh fly
(*Sarcophagidae*)

Bot fly (*Oestridae*) (Source:
http://www.cdc.gov/parasites
/myiasis/)

DIAGNOSIS: CUTANEOUS MYIASIS

Answer and Disease Summary

Etiology

- Larvae (maggots) stages of dipterous flies
  - Blow flies: *Calliphoridae*
  - Bot flies: *Oestridae*
  - Flesh flies: *Sarcophagidae*.

Source and Transmission

- Myiasis flies breed once in their life and the life cycle is usually concluded in 21 days. Gravid females lay batches on edge of a new wound.
- Larvae hatch, creep into the wound and dig, feed, and live in the tissue. Full-grown larvae leave the wound, drop, and burrow in the soil to pupate.
- The pupal survival depends on temperature; freezing or low soil temperatures (8°C) destroys this stage of the fly.

Occurrence

- All around the world
- Human and domestic mammals.

Clinical Findings and Lesions

- Adult flies deposit eggs on the body of the host.
- Eggs are glued to hairs.
- The eggs hatch in several days and penetrate the skin.
- Infestation of tissue with fly larvae (maggots), which feed on the host's dead or living tissue results in tissue inflammation.
- Such invasions can be benign in effect but others may result in a variety of conditions, including death.

Differential Diagnosis

- Cutaneous hypodermiasis.

Treatment

- Systemic ivermectin or organophosphorous insecticides in various formulations are effective:
  - Avermectins and Milbemycins
    - Avermectins abamectin, doramectin, eprinomectin, ivermectin, milbemycins, moxidectin. and selamectin. Ivermectin is the most commonly used and widely available.

- Organophosphate insecticides
  - Organophosphates used topically include coumaphos, diazinon, dichlorvos, famphur, fenthion, malathion, trichlorfon, stirofos, phosmet, and propetamphos.
- Dressing of wounds: debridement, drainage, removal of foreign bodies, and washing of lesions with antiseptic solutions.
- Antibiotic application to severely damaged areas prevents secondary infections.

Control and Prevention
- Improve hygienic practices and limit exposure to flies.
- Larvae can be controlled by applying or dusting insecticides such as tetrachlorvinphos to the back. Treatment must be repeated every 30—45 days during the flies season to control newly appearing larvae.
- Insect repellents or isolation of animal from exposure to fly attacks.
- Traditional ethno-pharmacology in some communities in Africa uses plants such as *Aloe ferox*, *Prunus persica*, and *Phytolacca heptandra*. Also disinfectants and antiseptics as well as diesel and petrol are used.
- Dressing of wounds: debridement, drainage, removal of foreign bodies, and washing of lesions with antiseptic solutions.
- Antibiotic application to severely damaged areas prevents secondary infections.

Clinical Quiz No. 14

What is your diagnosis?

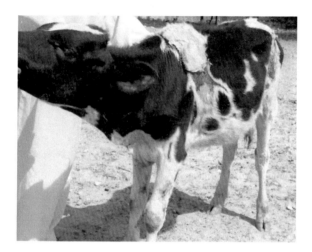

A calf (Friesian–Kenana cross) showing red inflamed severe lesions on skin, mainly on the white-colored (pale, unpigmented) parts. The skin cracks open, dries up, and large pieces of skin fall off leaving a sore patch underneath. Symptoms comprise photophobia from sunlight or the animal become nervous and seems uncomfortable, rubbing nonpigmented areas such as ears, eyelids, and muzzle. In the beginning lesions develop in hairless, white-haired, nonpigmented skin. Erythema progresses quickly and edema follows. Prolonged lesions increase to become vesicles with the exudation of serum, sores, scab formation, and even skin necrosis. In the late stages skin sloughing is a common outcome.

LABORATORY DIAGNOSIS

Specimen
- Liver biopsy
- Suspected toxic plants.

Skin Diseases of Cattle in the Tropics. DOI: http://dx.doi.org/10.1016/B978-0-12-811054-6.00014-3

Laboratory Tests and Findings

1. Liver function tests: liver enzymes and liver biopsy samples may be required to assess liver functions.
2. Identify poisons: find photodynamic agents in animal environment. Look for liver damaging poisons.

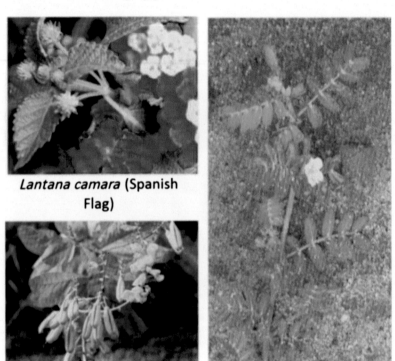

Lantana camara (Spanish Flag)

Crotalaria sp. (Rattle pods)

Tribulus terrestris (Devil's thorn)

DIAGNOSIS: PHOTOSENSITIZATION (PHOTOSENSITIVE DERMATITIS)

Answer and Disease Summary

Etiology

Photodynamic agents:

- Drugs (eg, psoralens, tetracyclines, fluoroquinolones, nonsteroidal anti-inflammatory agents, and amiodarone)
- Plants (eg, *Tribulus terrestris* (devil's thorn) and *Lantana camara* (ornamental garden shrubs))
- Other substances.

Source and Transmission

- Photosensitization occurs when animal forage poisonous plants that contain photodynamic agents and in animals with impaired livers.
- Intake of drugs or poisonous plants with photosensitizing properties and exposure to UV radiation increases the possibility of photosensitization, sunburn, and photo damage to the skin

Occurrence

- Worldwide
- Can affect any species
- Most commonly seen in cattle, sheep, goats, and horses
- In animals with liver damage associated with various poisonings (eg, *Senecio* spp.).

Clinical Findings and Lesions

- Photosensitization is a clinical condition in which skin (areas exposed to light and lacking significant protective hair, wool, or pigmentation) is hyperreactive to sunlight due to the presence of photodynamic agents.
- Lesions commonly seen on pale-colored (white) parts on the back and around nose but can happen anywhere.
- Skin become red and inflamed, then cracks open.
- Sometimes the skin dries up and large pieces of skin fall off leaving a sore patch underneath.

Differential Diagnosis

- Sunburn.

Treatment
- Prognosis in case of primary photosensitization is mostly good; nevertheless, hepatogenous photosensitization and porphyria has poor prognosis.
- Treatment generally includes supportive and palliative measures:
  - Dress wounds, cracks, and sore areas
  - Antibiotic application to severely damaged areas prevents secondary infections.
  - Corticosteroids, given parenterally in the early stages, may be helpful.
  - Secondary skin infections and suppurations should be treated with basic wound management techniques, and fly strike prevented.
  - The skin lesions heal remarkably well, even after extensive necrosis.

Control and Prevention
- Keep animal away from bright sunlight.
- Change pasture until you identify the source of poisoning. Or identify possible toxic plants and chemicals and remove from pasture.
- Fly control to prevent complications such as myiasis and cattle grub.
- Culling of breeds with photosensitization due to a genetic defect.

Clinical Quiz No. 15

What is your diagnosis?

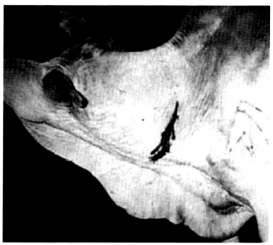

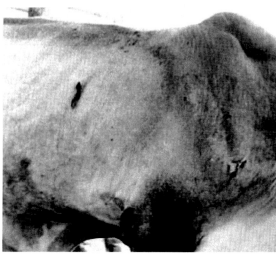

Bleeding and ulcerating skin from subcutaneous nodules in cattle. The lesions comprise circumscribed, hairless, slightly raised, dry, and hyperkeratotic areas. Lesions may ooze, cracking with scab formation. Skin lesions are commonly seen on the medial canthus of the eyes, the neck, sternum, and infrequently on the thorax and abdomen.

Skin Diseases of Cattle in the Tropics. DOI: http://dx.doi.org/10.1016/B978-0-12-811054-6.00015-5

LABORATORY DIAGNOSIS

Specimen
- Blood
- Exudates from lesions.

Laboratory Tests and Findings
1. Direct microscopy (Giemsa stain)

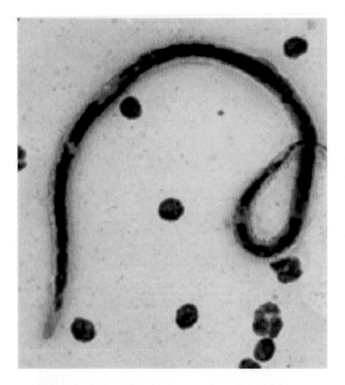

Microfilaria seen in a blood smear. Source: CDC, http://www.dpd.cdc.gov/dpdx/HTML/ImageLibrary/Filariasis_il. htmul5-02-9780128110546.

DIAGNOSIS: FILARIAL DERMATITIS (CUTANEOUS PARAFILAROSIS)

Answer and Disease Summary

Etiology

Microfilaria of *Parafilaria bovicola*

- Microfilaria is an early stage in the life cycle of parasitic nematodes in the family *Onchocercidae*.
- The adults live in tissues and circulatory system of vertebrates.
- They release microfilariae into the bloodstream of the vertebrate host.
- The microfilariae are taken up by blood-feeding arthropod vectors.
- In the intermediate host the microfilariae develop into infective larvae that can be transmitted to a new vertebrate host.

Source and Transmission

- The epidemiology of filarial worms is determined by temperature, rainfall, factors affecting the reproduction of vector flies.
- Following mating, female worms release microfilariae which are picked up by vector insects while feeding on host blood.
- Microfilariae molt and develop into infective larvae which are injected into the dermis layer of the skin.
- After 1 year the larvae molt twice into the adult worms.

Occurrence

- Tropical countries.

Clinical Findings and Lesions

- Blood-sucking flies and even house fly transmit the disease.
- Filarid worms form nodules in skin, lay eggs, and then microfilariae are released causing nodules to bleed and ulcerate.
- Although these lesions are inconvenient to the animal, ulcers heal spontaneously.

Differential Diagnosis

- Onchocerciasis
- Sporotrichosis.

Treatment
- No effective treatment is available.
- Topical treatment with ivermectin or organophosphorus compounds reduce the number and burden of parafilaria lesions.
  - Organophosphorus compounds such as Trichlorfon 6–10%, daily or on alternate days for 7 days, was found useful.
  - IVOMEC Pour-On at 500 µg/kg is indicated for the effective control of parasitic cutaneous infections including filarid worms.
- Secondary skin infections and suppurations should be treated with basic wound management techniques, and fly strike prevented.
- Surgical removal of debris and dressing of wounds is very efficient.

Control and Prevention
- Control of filarid worms focuses on decreasing microfilaria in blood and eradicating adult worms on skin and their vector flies.
- Vector control carried out by using environmentally safe insecticides applied by aerial spraying over breeding sites of flies is recommended. In some countries vector control is not feasible and costly.

Clinical Quiz No. 16

What is your diagnosis?

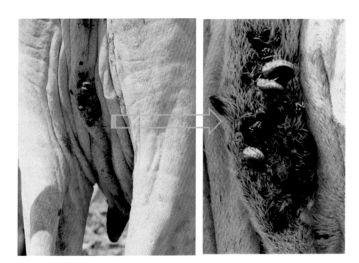

A cow infested with visible arthropod ectoparasites that were deeply embedded in the skin. Lesions are commonly seen inside legs, thighs, and udder regions. Lesions exhibit erythema, papule, intense pruritus, leaving thickened, wrinkled, skin with alopecia.

LABORATORY DIAGNOSIS

Specimen
- Collected ectoparasites attached to animal.

Skin Diseases of Cattle in the Tropics. DOI: http://dx.doi.org/10.1016/B978-0-12-811054-6.00016-7

Laboratory Tests and Findings

1. Identify ectoparasites: Find and identify ectoparasites (ticks) that are attached to animal.
2. Find ectoparasites: Check ectoparasites (ticks) in animal environment:

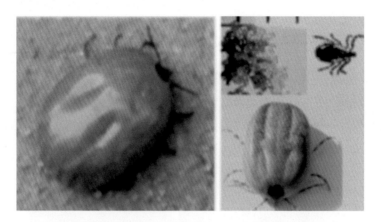

*Engorged adult female cattle ticks (*Boophilus *sp.) (left); numerous shiny golden eggs (top center); young tick (top right) and an engorged adult* Ixodes ricinus *(right bottom).*

DIAGNOSIS: TICK INFESTATION

Answer and Disease Summary

Etiology

Various genera including: *Amblyomma*, *Rhipicephalus*, *Hylomma*, *Ixodes*

- Ticks are ectoparasites (external).
- Ticks fall in the order Ixodida and along with mites they form the Subclass Acarina of the Class Arachnida and the Phylum Arthropoda.
- Ticks live on blood (hematophagy) of mammals, birds, and sometimes reptiles and amphibians.

Source and Transmission

- Prevalence of ectoparasites including ticks is higher in summer than winter and lower in rainy season.
- Malnourished cattle are susceptible to ectoparasitic infestation than animals with good conditions.
- Ticks flourish more in countries with warm, humid climates, because they require a certain amount of moisture in the air to undergo metamorphosis.
- Microclimate; as sandy soil, hardwood trees, rivers, and the presence of deer were found to increase tick populations.

Occurrence

- Worldwide in distribution but commonest in tropical and semitropical countries, especially where rainfall is high.
- The problem facing animal herders in both intensive and free range animals.
- Tick infestation is highest in Friesian, then the cross-breeds, and then the indigenous breeds.

Clinical Findings and Lesions

- Lesions inside thigh, neck, brisket, and tail
- Lesions are erythematous papules with intense pruritus
- Skin thickened, wrinkled, and alopecia appears
- Neglected sick animal condition deteriorates with anorexia, emaciation, and death.

Differential Diagnosis
- Mange
- Cutaneous hybodermiasis
- Cutaneous filariasis.

Treatment
- Affected cattle can be treated with a dip, spray, or other long-term acaricide drug. These treatments inhibit ticks from attaching to skin and may kill ticks that try to feed.
  - Systemic ivermectin or organophosphorus compounds
  - Topical organochlorine compounds and chlorinated hydrocarbons
  - Inspect animals and remove ticks by catching them with tweezers.

Control and Prevention
- Control of ticks in and around the home requires attention and treatment of both the outdoor and indoor environments, as well as attention and treatment of resident dogs and cats.
- Chickens and guinea hens provide an excellent natural source of tick control.
- Pasture Management: Ticks thrive on tall grasses. Pastures can be treated with a pesticide that kills ticks, such as permethrin.
- Reservoirs: Make fences and other measures to control wildlife such as deer and hogs from entering cattle pastures.
- Inspect new animal before admitting them into the pasture along with tick-free animals.

Clinical Quiz No. 17

What is your diagnosis?

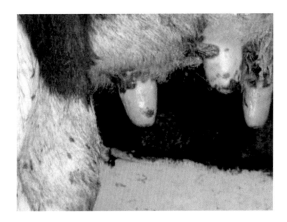

A cow showing ulcerative lesions on teats and udder. Lesions include vesicles with erythema which coalesce with wide oozing and sloughing of udder skin. Source: Dr. Colin D. Penny, Area Veterinary Manager, E Scotland/ NE England, Ruminant Business Unit, Pfizer Animal Health.

LABORATORY DIAGNOSIS

Specimen
- Infected tissue biopsy
- Blood sample.

Laboratory Tests and Findings
1. Tissue and blood
   a. Virus isolation
2. Blood (serum)
   a. FA (fluorescent antibody)
   b. Virus neutralization
   c. ELISA for antigen detection.

Skin Diseases of Cattle in the Tropics. DOI: http://dx.doi.org/10.1016/B978-0-12-811054-6.00017-9

DIAGNOSIS: BOVINE ULCERATIVE MAMMILLITIS (BOVINE HERPESVIRUS II)

Answer and Disease Summary
Etiology
Bovine herpesvirus-2

- Bovine herpesvirus-2 belongs to the family *Herpesviridae* (dsDNA) and is similar in structure to human herpes simplex virus.
- It causes bovine mammillitis and pseudo-lumpy skin disease.

Source and Transmission
- Bovine ulcerative mammillitis is often associated with cold weather.
- Commonly in early winter and in first lactation heifers.
- The virus is usually transmitted by direct contact between infected and susceptible animals during animal transportation and movement.
- Indirect transmission may occur via contaminated utensils and semen.

Occurrence
- It appears sporadically or in outbreaks.
- Young cattle are more susceptible.
- Massive outbreaks in milking cows with 30% morbidity.

Clinical Findings and Lesions
- Introduced by infected cows or biting flies, spreads via milking machines
- Incubation period 5–10 days
- Lesions on teats and udders
- Vesicles with erythema, coalesce with extensive weeping and sloughing of udder skin.

Differential Diagnosis
- Peracute staphylococcal mastitis
- Photosensitive dermatitis.

Treatment
- Treatment focus on curing of the skin and stopping the spread of infection to other animals.
- Dip teats with iodine-based dip or crystal violet lotion.
- Ointment and udder cream applied before milking soften scabs and speed healing of skin.
- Cannulation may be needed to ease milking.

Control and Prevention
- Separate and milk affected cows last.
- Udder wash and teat disinfection to reduce spread of infection.
- Disinfect milking machine and hands between cows and after milking.
- Check regularly to ensure that skin damage does not proceed to mastitis.

GIEMSA'S STAIN

Principle and Use
Giemsa stain is used to differentiate nuclear and/or cytoplasmic morphology of platelets, RBCs, WBCs, and parasites.

Composition
Stock Solution
- Dissolve 3.8 g of Giemsa powder into 250 mL of methanol.
- Heat the solution from step 1 to $\sim 60°C$.
- Slowly add in 250 mL of glycerin to the solution from step 2.
- Filter the solution from step 3.
- The solution needs to stand a period of time prior to use.

Working Solution
- Add 10 mL of stock solution to 80 mL of distilled water and 10 mL of methanol.

Procedure
- Place a clean 1- by 3-in. glass microscope slide on a horizontal surface.
- Place a drop (30–40 μL) of blood onto one end of the slide about 0.5 in. from the end.
- Using an applicator stick lying across the glass slide and keeping the applicator in contact with the blood and glass, rotate (do not "roll") the stick in a circular motion while moving the stick down the glass slide to the opposite end.
- The appearance of the blood smear should be alternate thick and thin areas of blood that cover the entire slide.
- Place the film over a piece of paper.
- Allow the film to air dry for 30–60 min.
- This slide can be stained as thick or thin blood film according to needs.

- Clearly label the slide.
- Wait for the film to completely dry
- Fix it by dipping the slide into absolute methanol, and allow the film to air dry in a vertical position.
- Stain the entire slide with diluted Giemsa stain (1:50, vol/vol) for 50 min (for a 1:50 dilution, add 2 mL of stock Giemsa to 40 mL of buffered water in a Coplin jar).
- Place the slide in the stain, *thick film down* to prevent the debris caused by dehemoglobinization from falling onto the thin film.
- Rinse the thin film by briefly dipping the film in and out of a Coplin jar of buffered water (one or two dips).
- Wash the thick film for 3−5 min. Be sure that the thick film is immersed but *do not allow the water to cover any part of the thin film.*
- Let air dry in a vertical position, then examine.

Results
Parasitic organisms (eg, malaria): the cytoplasm stains blue and the nuclear material stains red to purple. The sheath of microfilariae may or may not stain with Giemsa, but the body appears blue to purple.

GRAM'S STAIN

Use
Detection of gram-positive and gram-negative bacteria as well as yeast elements in tissue and smears from cultures. This is an essential stain and should be used whenever bacteria or yeasts are suspected.

Method
- Saturate a dry fixed smear with crystal violet for 1 min, and then rinse with water.
- Saturate the smear with iodine for 1 min, rinse again.
- Decolorize with gram decolorizes (acetone/alcohol) for 20 s, and rinse.
- Counter stain with safranin for 1 min, rinse.
- Carefully blot the slide dry with bibulous paper and observe under the microscope. Gram + stain purple; gram − stain red/pink.
- Negative specimens should be kept and reexamined the next day.

HEMATOXYLIN AND EOSIN STAIN

Use

The hematoxylin and eosin stain (H&E) is the most widely used stain in histology and histopathology laboratories. It has the ability to demonstrate a wide range of normal and abnormal cell and tissue components and yet it is a relatively simple stain to carry out on paraffin or frozen sections.

Preparation

- Acid Ethanol: 1 mL concentrated HCl + 400 mL 70% ethanol
- Hematoxylin: Harris hematoxylin with glacial acetic acid
- Eosin: Eosin Phloxine stain, working
- Permount: Histological mounting medium.

Procedure

- Stain rehydrated sections in Hematoxylin solution for 20−40 min.
- Wash in tap water for 1−5 min, until sections turn blue ("bluing").
- Differentiate sections in 70% ethanol—containing 1% HCl—for 5 s. This removes excess dye, allowing nuclear details to emerge.
- Wash 1−5 min in tap water until blue.
- Stain in Eosin solution for 10 min.
- Wash 1−5 min in tap water.
- Dehydrate, clear and mount.

Results

- Collagen: pale pink
- Muscle: deep pink
- Acidophilic cytoplasm: red
- Basophilic cytoplasm: purple
- Nuclei: blue
- Erythrocytes: cherry red.

POTASSIUM HYDROXIDE (10% KOH)

Use

For the direct microscopic examination of skin scrapings, hairs, nails, and other clinical specimens to see fungal elements.

Preparation

- Dissolve 10 g KOH in 90 mL water, mix and then add 10 mL glycerol, mix gently. 20% KOH is also used, it can be prepared by dissolving 20 g KOH in 90 mL water, mix and then add 10 mL glycerol, mix gently.

Making mounts for microscopy:

- Using an inoculation needle remove a small portion of the specimen, especially from any necrotic or purulent areas, and mount in a drop of KOH on a clean microscope slide.
- Cover with a coverslip, squash the preparation with the gentle pressure.
- Blot off the excess fluid.
- Gently heat by passing through a flame two or three times. Do not boil.
- Wait 20 min for skin scrapings to several hours for nail scrapings (specimen cleared).
- Examine microscopically for the presence of "refracting" fungal elements.

Note: negative specimens should be kept and reexamined the next day to avoid reporting false-negative results due to delayed clearance and staining of the specimen.

POTASSIUM HYDROXIDE (10% KOH) WITH PARKER INK

Use

This stain is the same as 10% KOH but the addition of parker ink enhances the visibility of fungal elements. For the direct microscopic examination of skin scrapings, hairs, nails, and other clinical specimens to see fungal elements.

Preparation

- Dissolve 10 g KOH in 80 mL water, mix and then add 10 mL glycerol and 10 mL Parker ink permanent blue ink then mix gently.

Making mounts for microscopy:

- Using an inoculation needle remove a small portion of the specimen, especially from any necrotic or purulent areas, and mount in a drop of KOH on a clean microscope slide.

- Cover with a coverslip, squash the preparation with the gentle pressure.
- Blot off the excess fluid.
- Gently heat by passing through a flame two or three times. Do not boil.
- Wait 20 min for skin scrapings to several hours for nail scrapings (specimen cleared).
- Examine microscopically for the presence of faintly blue stained fungal elements.

Note: negative specimens should be kept and reexamined the next day to avoid reporting false-negative results due to delayed clearance and staining of the specimen.

LACTOPHENOL COTTON BLUE

Use
For the staining and microscopic identification of fungi from cultures.

Preparation
- Cotton Blue (Aniline Blue) 0.05 g; Phenol Crystals (C6H5O4) 20 g; Glycerol 40 mL; Lactic acid (CH3CHOH COOH) 20 mL; Distilled water 20 mL.

This stain is prepared over 2 days:

- On the first day, dissolve the Cotton Blue in the distilled water. Leave overnight to eliminate insoluble dye.
- On the second day, wearing gloves add the phenol crystals to the lactic acid in a glass beaker. Place on a magnetic stirrer until the phenol is dissolved.
- Add the glycerol.
- Filter the Cotton Blue and distilled water solution into the phenol/glycerol/lactic acid solution.
- Mix and store at room temperature.

INDIA INK

Use
To demonstrate the capsule which is seen as an unstained halo around the organisms distributed in a black background. This is employed for fungal diagnostics especially for *Cryptococcus neoformans*.

Preparation

- Black charcoal ash (pulverize); Distilled water, Glycerol or gelatin; vinegar.

  Homemade preparation of India ink:

- Place the charcoal ash in the small bowl.
- Add water slowly and stir with a hard bristled brush until the charcoal dissolves.
- Add a few drops of vinegar and mix thoroughly to create stability in the ink once it has dried.
- Place the ink in a tightly lidded jar.
- Ink is now ready to use.

Procedure

- Place a loopful of India ink on the side of a clean slide.
- A small portion of the solid culture is suspended in saline on the slide near the ink and then emulsified in the drop of ink, or else, mix a loopful of liquid culture of specimens like CSF with the ink.
- Place a clean cover slip over the preparation avoiding air bubbles.
- Press down, or blot gently with a filter paper strip to get a thin, even film.
- Examine under dry objectives followed by oil immersion.

FURTHER READING

Blood, D.C., 1999. Pocket Companion to Veterinary Medicine, ninth ed. A Saunders Ltd.

Hamid, M.E., Mohamed, G.E., Abu Samra, M.T., El Sanousi, S.M., Barri, M.E., 1991. Bovine farcy: clinico-pathological study of the disease and its etiologic agents. J. Comp. Pathol. 105, 287−301.

Hamid, M.E., Kheir All, K.M.S., Ahmed, S.S., El Shiekh, A.E., Ibrahim, K.E.E., 2006. Unusual manifestation of a concurrent demodectic and sarcoptic mange in a Zebu-Friesian cross-bred heifer: clinical communication. J. S. Afr. Vet. Assoc. 77, 90−91.

Kahn, C.M. (Ed.), 2010. Merck Veterinary Manual, tenth ed. Merck & Co., Inc., Whitehouse Station, NJ.

Kampa, J., 2006. Epidemiology of Bovine Viral Diarrhoea Virus and Bovine Herpesvirus type 1 Infections in Dairy Cattle Herds (Doctoral thesis). Swedish University of Agricultural Sciences, Uppsala.

Quinn, P.J., Carter, M.E., Markey, B.K., Carter, G.R., 1999. In: Quinn, P.J. (Ed.), Clinical Veterinary Microbiology. Wolfe, Baltimore, MD.

Radostits, O.M., Gay, C.C., Hinchcliffe, K.W., Constable, P.D., 2007. Veterinary Medicine, tenth ed. W.B. Saunders Co, Philadelphia, PA.

The Cattle Site—Cattle Health, Welfare and Diseases News5m Publishing, Benchmark House, 8 Smithy Wood Drive, Sheffield, S35 1QN, England. http://www.thecattlesite.com.

Tiberg, K., 2011. http://classes.uleth.ca/201101/biol4800a/student%20presentations%20II/karma.ppt.

INDEX

A

Abrasion, 43
Abscess, 49, 51, 57
Acarina, 71
Acid-fast, 38, 42
Actinomyces bovis, 33–34
Actinomyces spp., 34
Actinomycete, 6, 39
Actinomycosis, 34, 40, 43
Agro-climates, 47
Alopecia, 69, 71
Amblyomma, 71
Anaerobic culture, 32
Anaerobic, 6, 34
Animal herders, 71
Arthroconidia, 10
Arthropod parasite, 20, 24
Aspirate, 32, 38, 41

B

Besnoitasis, 7, 21
Besnoitia besnoiti, 17
Biopsy, 3, 15, 19, 28, 32, 37, 41, 46, 50, 61–62, 73
Bite wounds, 43
Biting flies, 17
Biting insects, 6
Biting-fly population, 47
Bleeding, 65
Blood, 4, 6, 9, 28–29, 32, 45–47, 66–67, 71, 73, 77
Blood, D.C., 83
Blood agar, 4, 32
Blood smear, 66, 77
Bony swellings, 31
Bot flies, 59
Bovine besnoitiosis, 17
Bovine farcy, 39, 43, 83
Bovine herpesvirus-2, 74
BPV, 29
Bradyzoites, 16–17
Branching filamentous, 33, 38
Branching filaments, 4–5, 39

C

Calliphoridae, 59
Capripoxvirus, 47

Cheesy pus, 39, 51
Chronic skin infection, 3
Cigar shape, 50
Colonies, 6, 32, 38–39, 42
Communal grazing, 47
Contaminated environmental materials, 21, 25
Contaminated utensils, 74
Cord-like, 37
Cracks, 64
Cross breeds, 71
Crust, 3, 7, 9–10, 12–13, 19, 23, 26, 47
Cryptococcus neoformans, 81
Cysts, 16–17

D

Deformation, 31
Demodectic mange, 51
Demodex bovis, 25, 51
Demodicosis, 51
Dermatitis, 9, 12, 19–21, 23, 25, 51, 55, 67, 74
Dermatobia hominis, 55
Dermatomycoses, 7
Dermatophilosis, 6, 12, 21, 25, 29
Dermatophytes, 12
Devil's thorn, 63
Diptera, 53
Direct microscopic examination, 79–80
Direct microscopy, 10, 20, 24, 32, 38, 41, 50, 66
Discharge, 32, 34, 38–39, 41, 50
Discharging pus, 43

E

Ectoparasites, 69–71
Edema, 17
EDTA, 46
Electron microscopy, 28
Elephant skin disease, 17
ELISA, 28, 46, 73
Enlargement of superficial lymph nodes, 17
Eosinophilic intranuclear inclusions, 46
Epidermophyton, 12
Erythema, 69, 71, 73–74
Exudate drainage, 31
Exudates, 66
Exudation, 61
Exudative dermatitis, 3, 6, 15

Printed in the United States
By Bookmasters